ISBN: 979-8-218-02896-1

Library of Congress Cataloging-in-Publication Data

Library of Congress Control Number: 1-11458184071

Printed in the United States of America

First printing edition 2022.

- Cover design by Royal Love Designs
- Edited by Beau Book Editorial
- Interior Design by Jerra Latrice (Gifted with a Pen)

This is a work of nonfiction. No names have been changed, no characters invented, no events fabricated.

OUR HEALTH, OUR TRUTH

A Conversation on Black Health and Wellness: Mental Health Crisis

NANDY SMITH, MPH

ACKNOWLEDGEMENT

I must start by thanking God. Thank you for loving me so.

I want to thank my parents, Marie and Clezier Smith. Mom and dad thank you so much for supporting and encouraging me while obtaining my Master of Public Health degree.

I want to thank my family for always believing in me.

I want to thank my professors at Robert Stempel College of Public Health and Social Work at Florida International University. Educators are superheroes!

I want to thank my classmates. Study buddies, we did it!

I want to thank all the healthcare professionals; the world needs you.

I want to thank my daughter Legacy; you inspire me daily.

And to the Black community, you're worthy of living a healthy, quality of life.

Table of Contents

1
CHAPTER

BLACK HEALTH MATTERS

The health of African Americans in the U.S. hasn't always mattered. The aftermath of racism is felt today through systemic racism. Systematic racism has caused health gaps and set the foundation for poor health. The effects of slavery have infiltrated and shaped health conditions. The injustice experienced within the health care industry is a form of oppression for the black community. For black health to truly matter, the elimination of health care disparities should be a priority.

The health of African American seems to always take a toll for the worse with almost all diseases. At the beginning of the COVID-19 pandemic, there were conspiracies that black people could not catch the coronavirus. It was said that black people were immune from the virus. We, unfortunately, learned quickly that was a myth. The black population has disproportionally suffered the effects of COVID-19 more than any other racial group in the U.S. However, the concept of black people being immune from a disease is nothing new.

In 1793, a pandemic broke out in Philadelphia that killed thousands of the city's populations. Yellow Fever was a mosquito-spread virus that caused the skin and eyes to turn yellow. This is called jaundice.

The wealthy residents fled the cities to the country for protection. This was very similar to what occurred during the COVID-19 pandemic. During the Yellow Fever pandemic, doctors believed African Americans were immune. Physicians believed biological differences based upon race meant black people could not contract the virus. As a result, black nurses were expected to tend to the white population. It turned out that black people were not immune to the deadly virus, but by then, it was too late. They fell ill and died from exposure to the Yellow Fever just as the white population did.

These examples are important to remember because they represent the lack of care and lack of protection for the black community within the health industry. The black community has not been a priority. The belief that black people do not feel pain, or they can endure more pain than whites, stemmed from slavery. The inequalities of the health system are not a new theory in the U.S. Today, the environment and poor living conditions of the black communities make individuals more vulnerable to diseases. It's the same concept, but a different era. The mortality rate of black people due to lack of access to health services has always been on the rise. Let's talk about health disparities while we're on the topic of imbalanced access to health services.

Health Disparities Among African Americans

The Centers for Disease Control and Prevention (CDC) identifies health disparities as "preventable differences in the burden of disease, injury, violence, or opportunities to achieve optimal health that are experienced by socially disadvantaged populations." Health care disparity is a common theme for African Americans, and we don't recognize it's a problem. Some disparities that hinder African Americans from living a healthy life are poverty, inadequate access to health care, and the environment.

Poverty

Poverty is a contributing factor to stress, death, and disease. And poverty is a major problem in Black communities. It's no secret that wealth provides access to all kinds of opportunities in America. Economic stability means an individual can afford healthy food, housing, health care, stability, and have a sufficient income to meet their basic needs. Unfortunately, wealth for black households compared to whites are unequal. Although the U.S. is the wealthiest nation, African Americans are disproportionately more economically insecure.

According to Statista, "In 2020, 19.5 percent of black people living in the United States were living below the poverty line. This is compared to 8.2 percent of White people." Less wealth translates to fewer opportunities, low-income levels, less savings, and less access to stable employment that may eventually lead to poorer health conditions. Another factor is that black people are more likely to be underemployed or underpaid. As a result, the median household income for black households is significantly low compared to any other ethnic group.

The disparities that exist today between the Black-White wealth gap can be traced back to slavery. White people were allowed to profit from the bodies of enslaved people. As a result, black people were not allowed to build wealth that caused a domino effect with future generations. The Great Recession in 2007 has made it difficult for the black community to close the wealth gap. Black households have fewer personal savings for emergencies, which puts them in a position to miss payments for important expenses such as medical and housing.

Inadequate Access to Health Care

As mentioned earlier, inadequate access to health care is a problem experienced in the black community. Inadequate access to health care may be caused by a lack of health care insurance. The price you pay for insurance usually offsets the price for a great doctor who provides quality care at a facility that can support and provide health services. However, without insurance, patients will have to pay out of pocket for quality health care. With the current high price of health care and no insurance, people are less likely to receive the care needed to maintain, heal, or prevent illnesses and diseases such as diabetes, hypertension, and cancer. This is a problem within the African American community.

Health insurance improves availability of monitoring health conditions and access to vital services that lead to preventative care. Every person should have it to help them live a healthy life, but the black community struggles to obtain it. One factor for not having health insurance is unemployment. When compared with other ethnic communities, the black community has a high rate of unemployment, which has been the main source of obtaining health insurance. This is a cycle that leads to inadequate access to health care. Underemployment can be another factor why African Americans do not have health insurance. Underemployment describes people who find work that is short-term. Part-time work, seasonal work, or work for only one day more than likely do not provide benefits such as health insurance, 401 (k), or paid time off (PTO).

The Affordable Care Act—better known as Obama Care—has created more opportunities for everyone to obtain health insurance they can afford. With this access, more individuals can receive the quality care they need. However, access to money to pay for affordable insurance may still be a barrier to care for some. Other barriers to quality health care range from unreliable transportation, a shortage in available doctors, and only certain insurances being accepted at a health care facility.

Neighborhood and Built Environment

Our environment—what we see and don't see, how and where we live, who we see, and what we do—play a major role in our health. When neighborhoods lack the things that are important for health, members in the community don't have the opportunity to break the cycle of being unhealthy.

For African Americans who live on a low income and who may live in impoverished neighborhoods, may be affected negatively by their surroundings. In most low-income areas, there are either no hospitals or hospitals that are not fully equipped and staffed to give quality care. Access to healthy options at neighborhood grocery stores are slim to none. Low-income neighborhoods are riddled with fast food restaurants. Parks, trees, and walking trails are non-existent to encourage exercising outdoors and an overall active lifestyle. Violent crimes are committed, lack of food is present within homes, and people who are homeless influence our health mentally, emotionally, and physically.

The very things they lack has been proven to be beneficial to maintain a healthy life. It doesn't have to stay that way because it can exist. Black communities can rally, support, and speak up for change in their neighborhoods by building the environment they need. Trees can be planted. Walking trails can be created. Quality hospitals can be erected. Medical training programs can be provided. Quality housing can be built. A better and healthier life is around the corner.

2

CHAPTER

DISEASES THAT DISPROPORTIONATELY AFFECT AFRICAN AMERICANS

According to the U.S. Department of Health and Human Services Office of Minority Health (OMH), black Americans are more likely to be affected by diabetes, heart disease and stroke, HIV/AIDS, cancer, asthma, pneumonia, and sickle cell anemia. In most cases, these diseases are found disproportionately more in the black community than in any other race or ethnic group. The environment, economic, and social factors play a role in the healthcare of African Americans. If you live in an unsafe neighborhood or home, it leads to stress and fear. If you are living in poverty, you are unable to afford to pay to see a doctor, pay for tests, and pay for prescribed medication. If you encounter disrespect, racism, or bullying, your mental health will decline. There is a false narrative that individuals know how to detect the signs and symptoms associated with a certain disease. The reality is the majority do not know what the signs and symptoms are to detect them. As a result, early warning signs are not recognized, leading to the progression of disease and difficulty reversing or treating it.

However, with early detection and proper care, most of the diseases are preventable. The major aspect of bringing awareness is informing people about what causes certain diseases. Improving health within the black community begins with it. So, let's start now.

Diabetes

Your body produces blood glucose, often called blood sugar, which is the body's main source of energy. When blood glucose gets too high, it may lead to diabetes. There are two types of diabetes. Type 1 diabetes is when your body cannot produce insulin. Type 2 diabetes is when your body can produce insulin, but your body does not favorably respond to it. Diabetes can lead to seriously high blood sugar levels that may lead to serious health problems such as end-stage kidney disease and limb amputations. African Americans have a higher risk of developing type 2 diabetes than white people and are twice as likely to die from it.

The signs and symptoms of type 2 diabetes often develops slow and over a long period of time. You can be living with type 2 diabetes with no obvious signs and symptoms. Here are the signs and symptoms for type 2 diabetes:

➢ Increased sensation of thirst.
➢ An increased desire to urinate.
➢ Increased hunger.
➢ Unexplainable weight loss.
➢ Consistent blurred vision.
➢ Frequent infections.
➢ Numbness or tingling in the hands or feet.

- ➤ Feeling overwhelmingly tired or fatigued.
- ➤ Areas of darkened skin, usually in the armpits and neck.

There is hope! Uncovering your family's health history is the first step in being aware. If your family has a history of obesity, then you know there is a higher possibility of you developing diabetes. While there is no cure for type 2 diabetes, it can be controlled with daily exercise, healthy eating, and losing weight. Other options for maintaining diabetes and keeping your blood glucose levels low are insulin therapy and prescribed medication for diabetes while under the care of a doctor.

Heart Disease and Stroke

The leading cause of death in the United States are heart disease and stroke. Coronary Artery Disease (CAD), which affects how the blood flows to the heart, is the most common type of heart disease. Someone who suffers from CAD has a greater risk of having a heart attack. In 2019, 360,900 people died from CAD. Of that number, African Americans are at a greater risk than Hispanics and whites to succumb to CAD. The signs and symptoms of heart disease are:

- ➤ Heart Attack: Intense chest pain or discomfort, pain in the upper back or neck, indigestion, heartburn, desire to vomit or nausea, extreme fatigue, dizziness, upper body discomfort and shortness of breath.
- ➤ Arrhythmia: Feeling a fluttering sensation in the chest.
- ➤ Heart Failure: Fatigue, shortness of breath, swelling in the feet, legs, abdomen, ankles, or neck veins.

A stroke is caused when blood supply to the brain is blocked or when a blood vessel in the brain bursts. Every year, more than 795,000 people in the United States have had a stroke. About 610,000 of these are first or new strokes. African Americans suffer more strokes than any other group of people. The most common conditions that increase the risk of heart disease and stroke among black Americans are high blood pressure, obesity, and diabetes.

The best method to quickly identify when someone is having a stroke is the F.A.S.T. test. According to Centers for Disease Control and Prevention (CDC), F.A.S.T. can save someone's life when you:

Face: Ask the person to smile. Does one side of the face droop?

Arms: Ask the person to raise both arms. Does one arm drift downward?

Speech: Ask the person to repeat a simple phrase. Is the speech slurred or strange?

Time: If you see any of these signs, call 9-1-1 right away.

The signs and symptoms of stroke are:

> ➢ Paralysis or the sudden numbness in the face, arm, or leg, most often affecting one side of the body.
> ➢ Problem with speaking or difficulty understanding speech, slurring one's words or sudden confusion.
> ➢ Experiencing sudden trouble with eye vision, blurred in one or both eyes.
> ➢ Lack of coordination, balance, dizziness, and the ability to walk.
> ➢ Feeling sudden severe headaches, or loss of consciousness.

High blood pressure, also known as hypertension, increases the risk of heart disease and stroke. More than 40% of African Americans are more likely to have high blood pressure than non-Hispanic whites. The numbers are worse for black women who are 60% more likely to have high blood pressure. According to the National Stroke Association, preeclampsia—high blood pressure developed during pregnancy—may cause a stroke that leads to a higher death rate among women than men. High blood pressure may also develop earlier in life and is usually more severe. African American women have the highest rate of obesity or being overweight compared to other groups. Concern over obesity has grown over the years because it contributes to high blood pressure, high cholesterol, and diabetes. These conditions increase the risk of heart disease and stroke.

HIV/AIDS

Human Immunodeficiency Virus (HIV) is a virus that attacks the body's immune system. If HIV is untreated, it can lead to acquired immunodeficiency syndrome (AIDS). AIDS is a chronic condition that can cause death. Centers for Disease Control and Prevention (CDC) reports that African Americans are disproportionately affected by HIV. Forty-three percent of new HIV diagnoses are among African Americans, and those who are living with HIV are unaware of their diagnosis. Black women account for 59% of new HIV diagnoses.

There are several symptoms associated with HIV that vary from person to person. The type of symptom an individual has depends on what stage of the disease they are in.

Stage 1: Acute HIV Infection

Within two to four weeks of being infected with HIV, most individuals will experience a flu-like illness that includes the following symptoms:

- ➢ Fever.
- ➢ Chills.
- ➢ Rash.
- ➢ Night sweats.
- ➢ Muscle aches.
- ➢ Sore throat.
- ➢ Fatigue.
- ➢ Swollen lymph nodes.
- ➢ Mouth ulcers.

Stage 2: Clinical Latency

In this stage, most people do not experience any symptoms because the virus is multiplying at a low level. Without HIV treatment, people move into the "chronic HIV infection" stage for 10 to 15 years without treatment. Some individuals, however, move through this stage faster than others.

Stage 3: AIDS

This is the late stage of the disease. If you have HIV and you are not receiving HIV treatment, the virus will weaken your immune system and progress to AIDS. Symptoms of AIDS are:

- ➢ Rapid weight loss.
- ➢ Recurring fever or profuse night sweats.
- ➢ Extreme and unexplained tiredness.

- Prolonged swelling of the lymph glands in the armpits, groin, or neck.

- Diarrhea that lasts for more than a week.

- Sores of the mouth, anus, or genitals.

- Pneumonia.

- Red, brown, pink, or purplish blotches on or under the skin or inside the mouth, nose, or eyelids.

- Memory loss, depression, and other neurologic disorders.

Discussions about HIV and AIDS are the most uncomfortable and difficult topics to discuss with the general population and even more difficult within the black community. Cultural biases such as embarrassment, misinformation, discrimination, and homophobia lead to a higher risk for HIV in the African American community. Fear of judgement from family and friends and the stigma surrounding HIV and AIDS creates hesitation and prevents people from getting tested for HIV or from receiving treatment and preventative care. Although condom use is still the best method of protection against diseases and sexually transmitted infection (STI), eliminating the negative stereotypes is a step in the right direction. Creating a safe place to have open conversations about HIV/AIDS, can empower an individual and community to get accurate information, get tested, and seek treatment. Treatment for HIV can make the viral load undetectable, which means a person can stay healthy longer and prevent the transmission of the virus to their partners through sex.

Cancer Disparities in the Black Community

The U.S. has made significant effort against cancer with a decrease in death and an increase in survivor rate. However, cancer still affects African Americans disproportionately. According to the American Cancer Society, "Black people have the highest death rate and shortest survival of any racial/ethnic group for most cancers in the U.S." Black women were 40% more likely to die from breast cancer in comparison to white women, according to the Centers for Disease Control and Prevention (CDC). According to the U.S. Office of Minority Health, black men are twice as likely to die from prostate cancer and have a five-year cancer survival rate that is lower than non-Hispanic men. Diseases like cancer are killing African Americans at a fast pace. Eliminating socioeconomic disparities like education and income can prevent cancer mortality in the black community.

One of the main barriers is not having health insurance. Health care inequities affects an individual's overall health and their decision making. For many people in low-income poverty communities, they can't afford treatment without health insurance coverage. Everyone can't afford to miss work to get routine screening for cancer even if they believe something is wrong with their health. It may seem like common sense for most, but for people who are already struggling financially, they must choose between their health and income. Nine out of 10 people living in poverty will choose to go to work over their health. The healthcare system for cancer treatment is not tailored to low-income people. However, it's imperative to recognize, listen to your body, and act quickly if something seems wrong.

Cancer Screenings-Early Detection

It is recommended that women 40 to 44 should consider breast cancer screening with mammograms (x-rays of the breast). Women ages 45 to 54 should get a mammogram every year, and 55 years and older every 2 years. The American Cancer Society states, "Women should also know how their breasts normally look and feel and report any breast changes to a health care provider right away."

Colon & Rectal Cancer & Polyps Screenings

Adults who are at risk of colorectal cancer should start screening as early as age 45 for colon cancer or precancerous polyps that can develop in the colon or rectum. This can be done with a stool-based test or a visual exam that looks at the rectum and colon. The American Cancer Society states that, "If you choose to be screened with a test other than colonoscopy, any abnormal test result needs to be followed up with a colonoscopy."

Cervical Cancer Screenings

Cervical cancer screening for women should start at the age of 25. Women under the age 25 do not need to be screened for cervical cancer since it's rare for this age group. it is recommended for women ages 25-65 to be tested for HPV (human papillomavirus) with a Pap test.

Lung Cancer Screenings

Individuals between the ages 50-80 who smoke frequently or have a history of smoking are at an increased risk for lung cancer. It is recommended they are screened for lung cancer annually.

Asthma

Asthma is a lung condition causing the airway to narrow, making it difficult to breath, cause a wheezing sound, and shortness of breath. Asthma affects people from all races, however, the risk for death and hospitalization for African Americans are much greater than any other ethnic group. According to the Office of Minority Health, black children were five times more likely to be admitted to the hospital than white children. One of the reasons is because African American children are more likely to have to low birth weight. The severity of asthma varies depending on the individual but oftentimes is triggered by dust, pollen, tobacco smoke, air pollution, pets, mold, and stress. For some people this condition is minor, while for others it can cause life-threatening asthma attack. Many black people living in urban areas are exposed to pollutants. Social determinants, inequities in healthcare, and genetics are associated with the disparities within African Americans. There is not a cure for asthma, but it can be controlled through treatment.

Symptoms of asthma can vary, and they can vary in severity. The most common symptoms include:

➤ wheezing when exhaling.

➤ shortness of breath.

➤ coughing.

➤ excess mucus production.

➤ chest tightness.

Pneumonia

Pneumonia is an infection in the lungs caused by bacteria, viruses, and fungi. The air sacs are filled with pus and liquid making it difficult to breath. Pneumonia is a serious infection that can cause severe illness in people. Preventive care for pneumonia is getting vaccinated, good hygiene practices, and healthy lifestyle changes. Also, manage and prevent medical conditions like diabetes, asthma, or heart disease. Signs and symptoms of pneumonia:

- ➤ Cough that produces mucus.
- ➤ Chest pain when breathing or coughing.
- ➤ Fever, sweating and shaking chills.
- ➤ Nausea and/or vomiting.
- ➤ Shortness of breath.
- ➤ Confusion in older individuals.

Sickle Cell Anemia

Sickle cell anemia is an inherited disease that affects the red blood cells. Red blood cells are round, flexible, and move through blood vessels with ease carrying oxygen to all parts of the body. When sickle cell anemia is present, the red blood cells are shaped like a sickle or crescent moon. Instead of moving with ease and flexibility, the red blood cells move slowly and can block blood flow. When the blood flow is blocked, oxygen to the rest of the body is blocked as well.

Sickle cell anemia affects black Americans with signs of the disease surfacing as early as 6 months of age. Symptoms vary from person to person, but some initial signs to look for when diagnosing sickle cell anemia are:

- ➢ Extreme fatigue
- ➢ Periods of intense pain felt at different areas throughout the body
- ➢ Swelling of the body
- ➢ Infections
- ➢ Stunted puberty or natural growth
- ➢ Vision issues
- ➢ Yellow tinted skin and eyes.

Due to a lack of oxygen flowing throughout the body, sickle cell anemia may cause other conditions such as:

- ➢ stroke
- ➢ acute chest syndrome
- ➢ pulmonary hypertension
- ➢ organ damage
- ➢ blindness
- ➢ gallstones
- ➢ leg ulcers
- ➢ pregnancy complications like high blood pressure and blood clots.

For women with sickle cell anemia who want to have children, should consider a genetic counselor before trying to conceive. A genetic counselor will help explain available treatments and preventive measures as there is a risk of passing the disease to your child, as well as the possibility of suffering a miscarriage and premature birth.

COVID-19

The COVID-19 pandemic has underscored the issue. Researchers noticed higher death and hospitalization rates for black people. The patterns persisted, with black patients being nearly two times as likely as whites to die of the virus and black men having the highest rate of COVID deaths.

Data from the Centers for Disease Control and Prevention indicate that black Americans are twice as likely to die of COVID-19, compared with white Americans.

3

CHAPTER

BLACK WOMEN'S MATERNAL AND INFANT HEALTH

Pregnancy, depending on the person, can be a time of joy, fear, uncertainty, or a mixed bag of emotions about creating a new life and bringing a child into the world. No matter the emotion surrounding the baby, pregnancy should also include the health and life of the child and soon-to-be mother.

Mental Health

Pregnancy and childbirth can be an exciting time for mothers, but it also comes with some challenges. Expectant and new mothers often struggle with mental health silently. Maternal mental health problems and maternal health can lead to maternal mortality and morbidity. Mental health issues such as anxiety, stress, and depression are common during pregnancy. There are some expectant mothers who experience more severe symptoms than others. After the child is born, the mother is susceptible to postpartum depression, a serious mental illness that affects your behavior and physical health. Symptoms of postpartum depression such as sadness, emptiness, and feeling unconnected to your baby can interfere with your day-to-day activities and last longer than two weeks.

Maternal mental health problems among pregnant women often go undiagnosed since the symptoms associated with pregnancy-related symptoms are similar. Symptoms such as fatigue, frequent crying, poor sleep, and mood swings are not alarming symptoms in pregnancy, therefore, it goes untreated. Some pregnant women with mental health behaviors may use alcohol and substance abuse. This increases their risk for complications and preterm birth. Maternal suicide and overdose are the leading cause of maternal death occurring within the first year of postnatal. The statistics often do not count suicide as a cause of death for maternal mortality. Instead, they are counted as medical complications. Health care providers fail to acknowledge the signs of depression during a woman's pregnancy checkups. The mental health of a mother has an enormous impact on the child's behavioral, emotional, and mental health. A pregnant woman's mental health may also impact the development of her child. Maternal depression is linked to low infant birth rate, malnutrition, infectious illness, high rates of diarrheal disease, and other severe complications for an infant. It also negatively influences physical, cognitive, social, behavioral, and emotional development of a child.

Types of Maternal Mental Health Disorders

- Depression /Postpartum Depression

  Symptoms of postpartum depression include:

  ➤ Crying more often
  ➤ Feeling angry

- ➤ Isolating from family

- ➤ Feeling numb, empty, or not connected to your baby

- ➤ Worrying about hurting your baby

- ➤ Feeling guilty about not being a good mother, or doubting your ability to be a good mother

- Anxiety Disorder

  Symptoms of anxiety include:

  - ➤ Feeling restless, wound-up, or on-edge

  - ➤ Being easily fatigued

  - ➤ Having difficulty concentrating

  - ➤ Being irritable

  - ➤ Sweating

  - ➤ Difficulty controlling feelings of worry

  - ➤ Having sleep problems, such as difficulty falling or staying asleep, restlessness, or unsatisfying sleep

How does maternal mental health specifically affect black women? According to the National Perinatal Association, between 20-25 percent of women suffer from perinatal mood and anxiety disorders (PMAD). However, black mothers are more likely to experience PMAD like postpartum depression than white mothers and less likely to receive treatment. Black mothers are more vulnerable to maternal mental health due to socioeconomic status and systemic racism. Some of the risk factors include gaps in health insurance coverage, access to high-quality medical care, financial barriers (income), education, environment, exposure to trauma, stress, and much more factors. These risk factors along with untreated mental health issues prior to and during pregnancy may lead to postpartum depression. Improving black maternal mental health issues begin with bringing awareness to public health.

Prenatal Care

Prenatal care is so important for the woman and child to successfully ensure a safe and healthy pregnancy. Prenatal care is the health care a woman receives while she's pregnant. It includes checkups from a doctor, nurse, or midwife that can help keep the baby and the mother healthy. It's also an early detection prevention method to detect health problems early. Multiple factors contribute to high rates of maternal and infant mortality as well as poor health outcomes for black women. Some of these disparities are obtaining quality health care, underlying chronic health conditions, income, education level, and racism. A hospital that predominately services African Americans may contribute to a woman's maternal complications because most hospitals located in minority communities often provide lower quality maternal care. Black women are less likely to have health insurance coverage prior to pregnancy. A pregnant woman who doesn't have health insurance often delays prenatal care in the first trimester until Medicaid kicks in. It's also important to mention that most pregnant women are not comfortable speaking to their Obstetrician-Gynecologists (OBGYN), even when they suspect something is wrong with their health. There is a lack of trust and communication in the patient-physician relationship in our community.

During pregnancy, women are at risk of gestational diabetes, preterm labor, infections, and other severe complications.

Complications during pregnancy, labor and delivery may also lead to death. Maternal and infant deaths affect all women regardless of their race or socioeconomic background. The United States has the highest rate of maternal and infant mortality than any other developed country. Almost 60% of maternal deaths are preventable, yet the maternal mortality rate continues to rise. Of this number, CDC reports that black women are three times more likely to die from a pregnancy-related cause than white women. Many black women stated their pleas for help were ignored and they were overlooked when they expressed feeling pain, even though they were more likely to experience preventable maternal death and illness. It's believed that medical staff tend to think black women can deal with the pain or they are being overly dramatic or complaining. The time to have a conversation about this is now to raise awareness about maternal and infant health for black women and their children.

Black Maternal and Infant Mortality

Racial and ethnic disparities is apparent in maternal and infant mortality in the U.S. African Americans have the highest rate of infant mortality. The infant mortality rate is 2.3 times higher in black infants than in non-Hispanics whites. Black babies are four times more likely to die from complications related to low birthweight than white babies. Preterm birth is a prime example of racial disparities in infant mortality. Preterm birth is when a baby is born before 37 weeks of pregnancy. It's important to understand that a baby needs to fully develop the brain, lungs, and liver in the final weeks. When a baby is born too early, that child is at a higher risk for development delay, vision and hearing problems, cerebral palsy, breathing problems, and death. Although other women of color like American Indian and Alaska Native (AIAN) and

Latina women also experience higher rates of maternal mortality, African American women face a higher risk of poor maternal health outcomes. Black mothers are twice as more likely to receive late or no prenatal care according to the CDC. A woman's health and prenatal care affects the child.

African American women have a much higher rate of preventable diseases and chronic health conditions such as diabetes, hypertension, and cardiovascular diseases. These health conditions affect both the mother and child's health. It makes having a baby more dangerous and at risk for long-term complications. Black women often experience complications throughout their pregnancies. Preeclampsia (pregnancy-related high blood pressure), eclampsia (a complication of preeclampsia characterized by seizures), embolism (blood vessel obstructions), and hemorrhage (an escape of blood from a ruptured blood vessel), were leading underlying causes of death among African American women. Fibroids, benign tumors that grow in the uterus and can cause postpartum hemorrhaging, is often found in black women than in white women.

Another factor that contributes to maternal mortality is the age of a woman. The older a woman is, the risk for negative birth outcomes and complications increase. We can't ignore the fact that health inequities exist in educational and social economic factors that contribute to these complications. A college-educated black woman was more likely to experience complications during pregnancy than women of other race or ethnicities with a high school education level. Chronic stress, racism, and discrimination are some factors that cause physical "weathering", which is premature ageing or bodies that are worn down for black women. Weathering is associated to poor health outcomes and high death rates from chronic conditions. Stress has been associated with pregnancy complications such as preterm birth, increasing the risk for maternal mortality for black women.

Maternal and infant mortality is a public health crisis that stems from a long history of racism. Although slavery was an institution that lasted for over 400 years and ended in 1863 in the United States, the lasting effect of it, especially in the way black men and women were treated are still felt today. This racism and low view of black people extended into the health care industry. Structural racism is discrimination within institutions that limit opportunities, resources, power, and well-being of individuals and populations based on race and ethnicity. Structural racism is the primary reason African American women receive such poor treatment and low-quality care.

For black women, racism experienced in health care is highly prevalent with pregnancy, labor, and delivery. It tends to look like brushing off a black woman when she's seeking help for pain. It's making her feel inadequate or less than during a routine office visit. It means ignoring when she says there's something wrong. Medical providers fail to create a safe, welcoming environment for black mothers to feel comfortable to speak up during a checkup appointment. Black women constantly feel devalued and disrespected by health care providers. Many medical providers have this misconception that African Americans are uneducated, poor, low-status, and difficult patients. All these stressors of racism along with other daily life problems affect an individual even more so in pregnancy. The stereotype of the "strong black woman" has a negative effect on black women's health. The idea that black women are strong enough to endure pain creates an insensitive awareness and neglects the burden of mental stress a black woman faces daily.

Serena Williams, a famous tennis player who won 23 Grand Slam titles was no exception to complications during and after childbirth. In a cover story for the magazine Vogue, Serena talked about her postnatal journey and shared how hospital employees ignored her concern when she experienced discomfort, something that didn't feel normal. The problem started when Serena began to have symptoms of shortness of breath the day after giving birth to her daughter by C-section. Due to her life-threatening history of pulmonary embolism, a blood clot that causes blockage of an artery in the lung, she immediately told the nurse about her symptom. Serena requested a CT scan and a blood thinner, but the nurse thought she was confused because of the pain medication. Doctors ignored her request and performed an ultrasound on her leg instead. The ultrasound revealed nothing, and they finally decided to undergo a CT scan. The CT scan showed small blood clots in her lungs. Her concern turned out to be pulmonary embolism for which she was immediately treated.

Stories like Serena is not uncommon for many black mothers who are consistently being rejected in the medical field. Too many black women are dying in America of preventable maternal mortality. CDC reported that approximately 700 women die each year in the United States because of pregnancy or delivery complications. Complications affect more than 50,000 women who deal with life-threatening, pregnancy-related complications annually. Serena Williams clearly shows that racism in medicine can affect anyone at any income level. Doctors, nurses, and hospitals need to do a better job protecting and saving the lives black mothers.

4

CHAPTER

BLACK MEN'S HEALTH

Structural racism, and particularly racism within the healthcare system, has also affected black men. No matter what history reminds us of, it should not prevent black men from putting their health first with regular visits to the doctor.

In general, most men do not want to hear there is something wrong with their health, which is why men are not proactive in taking care of their health. *Black men should go get tested!* It's extremely important for black men to make it a priority and to get tested early to determine what ails them. African American men often wait too long before talking to their doctor about their health concerns. Most of the time, they don't consult with a physician until the problem has worsened and they've developed serious health complications. This delay often makes it difficult to treat a disease as well as prevent it. The fear of knowing is holding back black men from seeking medical attention. This fear of knowing is the reason black men have the lowest life expectancy compared to other ethnic groups. Chronic illnesses that are preventable and treatable, such as diabetes, stroke, obesity, and heart disease, are often found in the late stages This contributes to the major reasons for the lifespan gap. Other factors that contribute to the high rates of mortality for African American men includes having unprotected sex, lack of exercise, unhealthy diet, drinking alcohol, smoking, and using illegal drugs.

Early detection and treatment are keys that can be lifesaving because treatment is most effective in the early stages of a disease. Annual physicals may detect an illness early and prevent it from becoming deadly. There are several barriers that may contribute to late detection and rare visits to a doctor. No access to health insurance, poor quality of care, high rates of incarceration, socioeconomic status, and racial discrimination affect the quality of health for black men.

According to the CDC, the following were the leading causes of death of black men:

➢ Heart disease.

➢ Cancer.

➢ Unintentional injuries.

➢ Homicide.

➢ Stroke.

➢ Diabetes.

➢ Chronic lower respiratory diseases.

➢ Kidney disease, septicemia.

➢ Hypertension.

Did you know?

Black men are 50% more likely to develop prostate cancer in their lifetime and twice as likely to die from the disease.

Prostate cancer is cancer that occurs in the prostate. Prostate cancer is one of the most common types of cancer. In the early stages of prostate cancer, an individual may not experience any signs or symptoms. When it has advanced, Prostate cancer may cause signs and symptoms such as:

➤ Trouble urinating.

➤ Decreased force in the stream of urine.

➤ Blood in the urine.

➤ Blood in the semen.

➤ Bone pain.

➤ Losing weight without trying.

➤ Erectile dysfunction.

According to the Black Men's Health Project, black men are:

➤ 30% more likely to die from heart disease.

➤ 60% more likely to die from stroke than non-Hispanic white men.

➤ 75% less likely to have health insurance than white men.

➤ Nine times more likely to die from AIDS.

It is believed that being educated allows for improved health. Better health leads to higher income with access to health insurance and a healthier lifestyle. Studies have shown that black men with college degrees have a longer life expectancy compared to those with a high school level education. However, obtaining an education does not save black men. Regardless of their status in society, racism has made it difficult for black men. Black men have always needed to fight to survive, to protect, and provide for their family. Living in high crime and impoverished areas places them at higher risk of cardiovascular disease, diabetes, and infectious disease. Stress, and embracing coping mechanisms such as smoking, being sedentary, and violence, typically leads to poor health. When your body is responding to stress, your adrenal glands release the hormone cortisol into your blood stream. Black men in America are stressed, and stress may lead to a decline in physical, emotional, and mental health. Unfortunately, the health of black men has never been a top priority or a concern in America.

The real issues affecting the health of black men—racial profiling, discrimination, and police brutality—are never discussed. A black man walking into a store seems like a crime in our society when he is constantly being followed or harassed. A black man walking alongside a white woman on the sidewalk is alarming with thoughts of fear that he might snatch her purse. The way a black man is perceived in America by the way he walks, talks, and dresses is a problem in our society. Young black men who are arrested at higher rates than young white men live in fear of the police. According to the CDC, homicide is the leading cause of death for African American youth aged 10-24. Black teens and young adults are at higher risk for the most forms of violence than white teens. Teens who are exposed to violence, especially gun violence, may influence their development, learning challenges, and difficulty coping with stress. Adverse childhood experiences, or ACEs, are traumatic events that happen in childhood, from ages one to 17, that negatively affect the health and well-being of youth, particularly black youth. These childhood traumatic experiences can lead to substance abuse, smoking, depression, academic difficulties, suicide, and poor health outcomes.

The health of black young adults is a serious public health problem that has long lasting effects on their mental and social health.

Racism is also seen in the health care system. As mentioned earlier, men do not typically make their health a priority. It may be attributed to the poor quality of health care received by black men. It's even worse than the care received by black women. Another contributing factor to the poor health of black men is the lack of representation in the medical field. The lack of black doctors in predominantly black neighborhoods make it uncomfortable for people to seek care. Black men are already traumatized by the treatment received from the hands of white men. A white male doctor may not be someone a black man will feel safe with and trust they will give them proper care and fair treatment, especially concerning their health. Historically, attention to the health of black men by white doctors tend to fall on the low end of the spectrum.

A topic that never comes up when discussing black men's health is his relationship with his significant other. Too often, being in a committed, healthy relationship is not associated with good health. Being married improves the life expectancy of both men and women above those that are unmarried. This may be because married people tend to have better emotional and mental health and less likely to engage in risky behavior. The social support of having someone to care for you when you are sick and take you to doctor appointments improves one's health. It doesn't necessarily mean being married or in a committed relationship exempts an individual from sickness and disease. However, when it comes to black men, women tend to act as an accountability partner and be on top of the men's health. The women in their lives may be the ones who push them to get the medical care they require. There is a health benefit in being in a healthy committed relationship, particularly in a marriage.

Another issue that is not discussed is that black men have the highest incarceration rate than any ethnic group. The poor treatment of black men in prison also affects their mental health and well-being as an individual. The trauma left behind by images of police brutality and misconduct may also cause physical health concerns for the black community. Grief for black men as victims and loss of their lives create trauma. The psychological trauma of experiencing police violence, threats, and verbal racial insults increase the risk of PTSD, anxiety, paranoia, substance abuse, and suicide.

Racial disparities in health have negatively impacted black men in America. As a result, they also have a shorter life expectancy, higher rate of suicide, disease, and homicide than white men. These all have a direct effect on the health of black men. We must address this public health crisis if we want to improve the health of the black population.

5

CHAPTER

MENTAL HEALTH CRISIS AMONG AFRICAN AMERICANS

Our world has experienced a mental health crisis now more than ever because of the COVID-19 pandemic. The pandemic caused us to face many challenges such as stress and overwhelm. People have dealt with unexpected grief and loss during the pandemic. While there are some who did not believe in the existence of COVID-19, others experienced panic. Regardless of an individual's opinion on the matter, the world has tried to contain it. Social distancing was a necessary public health action to help reduce the spread of COVID-19. However, isolation from friends and family caused depression, anxiety, and stress. Many people have sought professional therapists to cope with how they feel and find ways to normalize their lives as much as possible.

African Americans face more challenges that cause emotional distress and affect their mental health compared to non-Hispanic whites. Even with the COVID-19 pandemic, the African American community was hit disproportionately with homelessness, unemployment, and food security. This has increased the amount of stress and anxiety for African

Americans along with everyday racial discrimination. As mentioned in the earlier chapter, racism, discrimination, and inequity affects the mental health of African Americans.

According to the CDC, racial disparities in suicide make some groups at a higher risk. Although African Americans were 60 percent lower than the non-Hispanic white population to commit suicide in 2018, it is a present problem for blacks. The Office of Minority Health stated the leading cause of death for blacks in 2019 was suicide for ages 15 to 24. Black men were four times greater to die from suicide than black women in 2018. Living below the poverty level is the leading cause to experience mental distress that may lead to thoughts of suicide.

Local, national, and world events have added to mental distress. Police brutality, the senseless killing of black people, gun violence, political elections, and the global COVID-19 pandemic has wreaked havoc on the mental stability of everyone. These events have specifically affected the black community who are left feeling tired of fighting, frustrated, angry, and sad. Feelings of hopelessness can arise, believing life for black people won't ever improve, and ultimately lead to stress, depression, or wanting to end your life.

In times like these, talking to someone—a spiritual leader, family member, friend, doctor, or licensed therapist—will help you deal with the range of emotions you or someone you know is feeling. Holding it in and keeping it to yourself will not help you to heal. The truth is if you try to fight by yourself, you're going to get tired of fighting. You deserve to be here. Give it to God because he'll never get tired of fighting for us.

Poverty is another major contributing factor for mental health. According to the Health and Human Services Office of Minority Health, black adults living below the poverty line are twice as likely to report serious psychological distress. Financial stress destroys families and affects an individual's mental health. Everyone wants financial stability in life rather than living paycheck-to-paycheck. It's not always equal for black people. African Americans don't usually have a fair and equal advantage of not being in poverty. Those who live in poverty are constantly worrying about where their next meal is coming from. Will the lights be cut off this month? Will there be an eviction notice on the door when they get home? Is the neighborhood safe enough for their children to play outside? Will they hear gun shots or see violence tonight? These are some of the worries that people who live in poverty think about. Despite African Americans having the highest rate of mental illness, they have lower rates of mental health services such as prescription medications and outpatient services. African Americans don't often receive the proper care for mental health illnesses.

According to American Psychiatric Association's Mental Health Facts for African Americans, here are the following statistics:

Compared to whites, African Americans are:

- ➢ Less likely to receive guideline-consistent care
- ➢ Less frequently to be included in health research
- ➢ Less likely to use mental health specialists, but more frequently use emergency rooms or primary care
- ➢ Less likely to be offered either psychotherapy or evidence-based medication therapy

- Less likely to be diagnosed with mood disorder, but more frequently diagnosed with schizophrenia
- Physicians verbally communicate with black patients 33% less than white patients
- Black people with mental health conditions, specifically schizophrenia, bipolar disorders, and other psychoses, are more likely to be incarcerated.

African Americans are also less likely to speak up about their mental health conditions. People in the black community believe that mental health illness is a sign of weakness. Many of the stigmas or misconceptions comes from a lack of awareness and understanding that it is an illness. The negative attitudes and beliefs towards people who live with a mental health condition is the exact reason why individuals suffer in silence. People tend to feel ashamed to admit something is wrong with them for fear of being judged. This fear often prevents people from seeking the mental health treatment they really need. African Americans usually feel safer seeking support from their faith community rather than seeking a medical diagnosis. The church has always been a place of refuge historically for African Americans. An individual's faith and spirituality are an important part of a treatment plan for someone who suffers from mental health illness, and it helps with the recovery process. Although the church is a necessary part, it shouldn't be the only form of intervention. Seeking professional care when experiencing mental health challenges will be crucial in the healing process.

A serious mental health condition that affects the African American community's mental health is the term colorism. This condition is often overlooked and deemed taboo, but it's far from a myth. Colorism has a negative, long-lasting effect that is serious among African Americans, especially black women. Colorism is the practice of favoring light skin over dark skin. In society, light skin is associated with high value and superiority. Dark skin is viewed as less beautiful and aggressive. The preference for lighter skin tones is a result of slavery. During the enslavement of black people, slaves who were light skinned received preferential treatment. They were often children of the slave master who raped a black woman.

Colorism has divided families, friendships, and society. Even after slavery, the preference for lighter skin continued with behaviors like forming the "Blue Vein Societies," where only black people who were light enough to see the blue veins in their skin were admitted to certain clubs. The "Paper Bag Test" was used to determine if someone was allowed to attend church, social clubs, fraternities, and other organizations. If an individual was darker than the brown paper bag, they wouldn't be allowed entry. Today, colorism is still prevalent in our society, in the media, and within black culture. It's important to note that light skinned black people also face discrimination within the black community. There's a misconception that the lighter a person, the easier or better treatment they will receive in society. Although, it may be true for some, it's not the case for all light skin black individuals. Many light skin people face just as many challenges that are sometimes overlooked.

Black women and young black girls are especially at risk for colorism. The European standard of beauty—women with straight long hair, small nose, and lighter skin tone—is glorified in our society. These images can lead to self-hatred, a mental illness called body dysmorphia that obsesses over perceived flaw in appearance, skin bleaching, depression, and eating disorders. Colorism is a systemic issue that plagues the world and it's a direct result of racism. It is rooted in racism and has silently affected the mental health of the black community. Colorism impacts the mental and behavioral health of African Americans. Colorism affects a person's emotional, physical, and mental well-being. Colorism is tearing apart the black community and damaging the mental health of both men and women. Like mental health illnesses, colorism is not talked about enough in the black community. Therefore, people will continue to suffer in silence. We must create a safe space for people to feel comfortable to express their emotions without being judged or dismissed. There are amazing efforts that are being done to bring awareness on both issues, but we have a long way to go before we can move forward.

Mental health does not define who you are as an individual. It's not a sign of weakness, in fact one possesses great strength once they are not in denial. You can take control of the condition instead of letting it control you. We are the sum of everything that has happened to us in our lives. Black people have been through so much trauma and continue to face adverse challenges even more so today. In fact, it almost seems as if history wants to repeat itself with the blatant racism in our world. African Americans are forced to witness unarmed black people dying and being treated unjustly and witness the murderers be set free without justice for the families or community. This happens all while witnessing the privilege of a white person be set free when they commit a crime and not held accountable for their actions.

Many African Americans view political representation as a possible catalyst for increased racial equality. African Americans become very hopeful when there's a politician who appears to be ready for "change" to see the black community progress. Instead, black people must endure broken promises. Politicians are constantly using the "black card" to win black votes but, never intend to keep their promises to the black community once in office. African Americans have a mistrust of white society. The disappointment can affect a person's mental health. It can lead to depression, stress, or anxiety. Waiting for the "change" that never seems to come can take a toll on their mental health.

African Americans have endured a lot. Racial trauma, also known as race-based traumatic stress (RBTS), refers to the mental and emotional injury caused by encounters with racial bias and ethnic discrimination, racism, and hate crimes. The amount of trauma that black people go through every day, makes it almost impossible not to experience some form of mental health issue. Post-traumatic stress disorder (PTSD) is a mental health condition that can develop as a response to a person who has experienced any traumatic event. Black people have experienced trauma since the beginning of time, generation-to-generation. The problem is black people are not taught how to cope or address the issue properly. Mental health is a public health matter, but it's a long-time crisis for African Americans. To change the stigma, the community must collectively continue to make room for conversations about mental health acceptance. Mental health among African Americans is real and it's a serious problem. Thankfully, it's something we can overcome just like we do everything else together.

Self-Help Techniques for Coping with Mental Illness

Awareness: *Listen to your body, be aware of changes with your emotional, physical, and mental health.*

Acceptance: *Accept your condition, accept yourself, accept your truth.*

Seek: *Don't be afraid to seek professional help.*

Self-care: *Take care of your mental health (meditate, prayer, medication, etc.).*

Support: *Reach out and talk to trusted people who are able support you and be there for you.*

Educate: *Educate yourself on mental health disease, symptoms, and treatment. Knowledge is power.*

6
CHAPTER

BLACK YOUTH TRAUMA

Black youth mental health is an emergency. African American adolescents in America experience mental trauma and it's often not talked about. We often don't recognize the amount of trauma that black youth face daily in our society. African American adults sometimes won't recognize signs of trauma in their own lives because it has become a common way of life. For example, discrimination is something that African Americans have suffered for years. Although we will never truly accept the treatment of being discriminated, we're also not surprised by it. The world has tried to condition our minds into thinking it's a normal way of treatment living in America. African American adults are not shocked about the racism and hate in the world. It's been going on for so long that we know how to mentally deal with it for our sanity. We've done that for every aspect of our lives whether it's racism, poverty, or violence. African Americans do not associate these challenges with trauma. Most people bury their personal childhood traumas and never confront them.

It's not that simple for young black adults living in America to turn off the trauma they've experienced. Their mental health is under attack.

Most black youth will never seek therapy or treatment to talk about the effect of their trauma. This makes it difficult to properly cope with their feelings and sometimes this may lead to risky behaviors such as substance abuse, violence, and aggression.

Violence: According to CDC, black youth are at a higher risk for the most physically harmful forms of violence such as homicides, fighting that lead to injuries, and aggravated assaults compared to whites. Homicide is a leading cause of death for African Americans of all ages. In the U.S. most homicides occur among people 15-34 years of age. The disparities between black and white youth are due to poverty, racism, education, social and economic disadvantages that contributes to the high rate of violence. This mainly affects young black males who are at a higher risk of homicide violence than young black girls. Being exposed to violence at a young age can cause long-lasting mental and physical health problems. Exposure to violence is associated with increased delinquency, risky health related behaviors (substance abuse, sexual risk behaviors), chronic disease, premature mortality, and other serious mental health complications. Violence, such as shootings and fights, scares people to even come out in their neighborhoods. Children are being robbed of playing at the park, walking, bicycling, and using recreational spaces.

Poverty: Living in poverty and being poor have numerous negative outcomes that affects an individual. Poverty contributes to violence, poor mental health, and poor decision making that may lead to risky behavior. Poverty in the U.S. continues to affect black people the most, as African Americans remain disproportionately poor. African American adolescents are more likely to live in poverty and have a disadvantage with their health, mental, social, and physical well-being. There are families in America who cannot afford to live paycheck-to-paycheck because the income they receive is not enough. African American children growing up poor are at greater risk of drug use, mental health disorders, disrupted physiological functioning and depressed academic achievement.

Racism: Racial disparities is causing a rise in suicide among black youth. Children who experience discrimination tend to experience issues with mental health. The disproportionate burden of mental health disparities on black children and adolescents has a lot to do with racism. The suicide and depression rate among black youth is on the rise. Although the COVID-19 pandemic has impacted the mental health among black youth, racism is a major contributing factor. Society often believes that schools are a safe, race neutral environment for children. However, black youth typically experience racism at an early age while in school from their peers, teachers, and staff. School administrations do not always respond to the complaints of black youth in a timely manner. In most cases, their response comes too late.

Black adolescents internalize racial discrimination silently, which results in depression and other mental health illnesses. Black students are constantly being bullied and are facing racist slurs in and outside of school. The n-word is written on lockers, walls, and restrooms by their white peers. According to The National Survey of Children's Health (NSCH), black, non-Hispanic children, ages 0-18 years, have experienced individual/interpersonal racism. Studies have also shown that black children under the age of 13 are two times more likely to commit suicide. Black youth have the highest suicide mortality rate in comparison to white adolescents.

The constant harassment and racism have taken a toll on the mental health of black youth. Adolescents who experience negative racial discrimination at school encounter lower grades, isolation, low engagement, fights, mental health, racial stress, and trauma. Young adults who suffer discrimination about their bodies, race, age, sex, or appearance have a greater risk of long-term mental health problems. According to the study published in the Journal of Pediatrics, people who encountered discrimination frequently or at least a few times a month, were 25% more likely to be diagnosed with mental disorder and twice as likely to develop severe psychological distress. Black youth are still able to succeed in school despite having to deal with racism. However, the trauma often leaves behind a scar.

The discrimination black adolescents encounter in school is not only from their peers, but from educators as well. This is an issue that needs to be addressed. There are teachers, faculty, and staff who also participate in bullying black children. The racism is demonstrated through their actions of dismissing the complaint of a black child who reports being harassed. There are also people who use racial slurs towards a black youth. This can be very confusing and hurtful for a child who feels attacked from both their peers and from an adult.

Exposure to racism at a young age can lead to anxiety, stress, and Post Traumatic Stress Disorder (PTSD). Black youth who have been exposed to violent behavior are at a greater risk for PTSD. The younger a person is discriminated against, the more likely they are to experience mental health problems.

Almost every black child has seen or heard videos of black individuals being murdered and harassed by law enforcement in broad daylight. It's been broadcasted for the world to see it. Black youth who witnessed violent acts, such as their neighborhood being burned down, are often left feeling scared, angry, and perplexed. Protestors everywhere are demanding justice for innocent, black victims. It can be overwhelming seeing and living in a divided world as a young adult. As much as parents want to shield their children from these illnesses and experiences, racism is too evident in our society.

7

CHAPTER

DISTRUST OF THE MEDICAL SYSTEM AMONG AFRICAN AMERICANS

Studies show there's a lack of trust in the minority community. Black and Hispanic people have less trust in their doctors in comparison to white people, especially if they have lower income, less education, and are without health insurance. This is a huge concern in public health. The problem is the less trust people have in the medical system, the less they use the medical system. This makes it difficult for patients to get preventive care and treatments they need to stay healthy. This also means there is a delay in conducting routine screenings and wellness checkups.

In life, trust is an essential part in all relationships. When trust is gained, an individual is more likely to feel comfortable and confident in receiving advice from the important person. They are more likely to apply the advice to their life. Similarly, trust is the most important part in the doctor-patient relationship. It also influences the decision making for a patient to seek help early. Most people don't understand how crucial it is for a patient to have trust in their physicians and healthcare providers. An individual who trusts their doctor is more willing to talk about their health concerns and follow their advice.

Many African Americans don't trust their healthcare providers to act in their best interest regarding their health. The term "medically disenfranchised" refers to people with no access or inadequate access to a primary care physician. This is due to a lack of doctors in their area to care for them. Access to primary care is limited. Medically disenfranchised black people experience discrimination in the health care system. As a result of racial discrimination in the medical system, many black individuals stopped seeking care or won't keep their scheduled follow-up appointments. This is a major factor in the health disparities between blacks and whites. African Americans compared to white patients receive poor treatment from health care providers. Unfair treatment such as being dismissed, misunderstood, aggressive or unpleasant care occurs. To address this distrust of the U.S. healthcare system among the black community, we need to talk about the root of where the problem started.

Why Don't African Americans Trust the Health Care System?

African Americans have many reasons to be distrustful given the history of exploitation from doctors and medical researchers. Distrust in medicine and research has been a constant historical theme as minority individuals have been targeted and at the center of ethical controversies. Historically, African Americans faced discrimination and abuse by medical professionals. The long legacy of being used in medicine, without consent, has left many black communities in fear of trusting medical professionals. The lasting effect of black people being mistreated is the reason for many of the strained relationships between doctor and patient. It's a constant reminder of the horrific treatment black ancestors had to endure at the hands of medical professionals. It's not surprising that in 2022, there's still a disconnect and distrust between medical professionals and black patients.

The Tuskegee Syphilis Study. In 1932, the infamous Tuskegee experiment began. During this time there was no known treatment for syphilis, a contagious venereal disease. About 600 African American men from Macon County, Alabama were enrolled in this project to study the full progression of the syphilis disease. United States Public Health Service (USPHS) was able to recruit these black men by promising them free medical care. It's important to note that some of these black men had never seen a doctor before. So, the black men accepted without hesitation to participate in the project. Doctors from the USPHS only informed the participants that they were being treated for "bad blood", which refers to a variety of diseases. In 1947, penicillin was the recommended treatment for the syphilis disease. The researchers were able to convince doctors to not give the participants any treatment.

The black participants suffered severe health complications like blindness and even death from the untreated syphilis. The participants had their blood drawn and spinal taps conducted by the study's white medical staff. The problem was for 40 years adult black men were monitored for a disease and left untreated despite the availability of effective treatment. This was an inhumane act on African American men. The unethical study of the Tuskegee experiment was exposed in 1972 by Jean Heller of the Associated Press. It caused a public outrage forcing them to shut down the study. However, by then, several participants had died, many from syphilis-related causes. The Tuskegee experiment impacted African Americans and their trust in medical research.

Henrietta Lacks. In 1951, a woman name Henrietta Lacks visited Johns Hopkins Hospital after experiencing vaginal bleeding. The Johns Hopkins Hospital at the time was one of the few hospitals providing care for African Americans. A doctor discovered a large tumor in her cervix upon examination. Henrietta was a young black mother of five children. Medical records revealed that Henrietta began radium treatment for her cervical cancer. A sample of her cancer cell taken from a biopsy was sent to Dr. George Gey, a cancer and virus researcher. Dr. Gey collected cancer cells from all patients regardless of their race at Johns Hopkins Hospital. Every sample cell died at his lab except for Henrietta's cancer cells. Her cancer cells were unlike the rest of the sample cells because they would double every 20 to 24 hours. Her cells survived and reproduced. As a result, the nickname "HeLa" cells were the first immortalized human cell line.

The unethical racial issue with Henrietta Lacks' story is that her cancer cells were used for medical research without her knowledge or consent. The researcher shared her cancer cells with other scientists and used them for biological research. The HeLa cells have been used to study effects of drugs, viruses, infectious disease, modern medicine, and the growth of cancer cells without experimenting on humans. HeLa cells also helped to develop in vitro fertilization. Henrietta's cells were significant in the development of polio and COVID-19 vaccines. Henrietta's story demonstrates the racial inequalities that are rooted in the U.S. research and health-care systems. Even after her death, doctors and scientists failed to ask her family for their consent. Henrietta's privacy was invaded with the release of her medical records to the media and revealing her name publicly. Researchers who used Henrietta's cells without her permission represent a reoccurring theme of medical professionals continuing to disregard African Americans. However, it also represents the crucial role of African Americans in medical research.

James Marion Sims, MD. Dr. Sims was the most famous surgeon in the 19th century that developed surgical techniques for women's reproductive health. At a time when treating women was rare, Dr. Sims operated on women. He's responsible for the invention of the vaginal speculum, a tool used for dilation and examination. He also created a surgical technique to repair vesicovaginal fistula, a complication of childbirth that causes pain and urine leakage due to a tear between the uteri. The "father of modern gynecology" performed experiments on black female slaves without anesthesia. He experimented on Lucy, Anarcha, Betsey, and many unknown enslaved women. Studies show that he performed 30 surgeries on Anarcha alone, all without anesthesia. These enslaved black women underwent surgery without treatment to numb the pain. It's the racist notion that black people, especially black women, do not feel pain.

It's not a surprise that black people in the U.S have a disproportionately low rate in receiving the COVID-19 vaccine. COVID-19 is a disease that is disproportionately affecting black people in several countries. Yet, African Americans have the lowest rate of vaccination. African Americans vaccine hesitancy is rooted in the mistrust of a historically racist healthcare system. It's simple: most black people don't trust medical professionals. The fear is they might be used in some form of experiment like a guinea pig and treated like lab rats. Also, the lack of transparency with medical researchers appears as if they have something to hide. Historically, doctors and scientists have lied to African Americans keeping them in the dark about treatment, research, and health developments. What the medical community is experiencing from African Americans regarding COVID-19 vaccines is a direct effect to a well-known cause. African Americans now have the option to decide to participate freely in clinical research or other studies. This also includes taking the COVID-19 vaccine. It's now about regaining power over their lives and their communities.

Of course, there's pros and cons in every decision we make as individuals. African Americans have the highest numbers in vaccine hesitancy because of the historical mistreatment at the hand of doctors and researchers. This can hinder the black community and discourage many black people from educating themselves on vaccines in general. Many black people are not informed about the long process of vaccines being created before it's available to the world. The past trauma and mistrust may have contributed to many African Americans in being closed minded when it comes to being informed on the COVID-19 vaccination. Rightfully so, it's a pain that's rooted deep within African American people. It's going to take time for black people to completely trust medical professionals. The U.S. hasn't always been good to African Americans.

8

HEALTH PROMOTION AND DISEASE PREVENTION

"Health promotion is the process of empowering people to increase control over their health and its determinants through health literacy efforts and multisectoral action to increase healthy behaviors."
-World Health Organization (WHO)

"Disease prevention, understood as specific, population-based, and individual-based interventions for primary and secondary (early detection) prevention, aiming to minimize the burden of diseases and associated risk factors."
-World Health Organization (WHO)

Health promotion interventions delivered in barbershops and hair salons show promise of improving health outcomes among African Americans. Hair grooming is an integral part of social life for many African Americans. Utilizing barbershops and hair salons as sites for intervention delivery can improve the health of black people. As mentioned in this book, many individuals who are part of racial and ethnic minority groups don't trust their doctors or the medical community. The lack of trust in the medical system or doctors cause people to avoid seeking medical advice, treatments, or preventive care. Locating health interventions in local barbershops and hair salons in predominately black communities means introducing a new method of delivering health care to African Americans. It's time to take a new untraditional approach in health care interventions. Many African Americans will not seek medical advice or treatment from healthcare professionals or doctors in hospital settings. An intervention in the community barbershops and beauty salons is a step in the right direction in promoting good health.

Black barbershops and hair salons are staples in the African American community. It's a safe gathering place to share and be heard about community related issues. There's a built-in trust relationship between the barbers, stylist, and the client. Trust is the core foundation of those relationships. Most clients are repeat clients and have been going to the same barbers and stylists for years. Barbershops and hair salons have become an intimate place for personal sharing and emotional comfort. People have shared their most confidential information in these places. These environments are usually a positive, empowerment, atmosphere. The barbershops and hair salons in the black neighborhoods are essential places for African Americans. Clients are more likely to share their health concerns with their barbers/stylist than to seek medical advice from a health professional. This level of trust is what health care professionals lack from their patients. This is why health professionals have leveraged these relationships to bring care to a hard-to-reach demographic, especially among black men.

An experiment was done at a local barbershop to reduce high blood pressure in a high-risk population. During the research experiment, barbers were trained to check blood pressure for their clients. The results showed an increase of a patient's retention and lower blood pressure levels due to barbers encouraging lifestyle modification. Individuals were more receptive to the barbers than to the health professionals. This intervention is crucial because African Americans, especially black men, are less likely to get regular health checkups than whites. Also, high blood pressure disproportionately affects black people who are also more likely to develop complications of stroke and heart conditions than other races and ethnicities. Health professionals can visit the barbershop and hair salons to perform screening and educate the community on health promotion.

We've all heard the saying "health is wealth", and it's true. The greatest success in life is living a healthy long life to enjoy your loved ones. There are some things we can do to prevent diseases and to take care of yourself.

Healthy habits to help prevent diseases:

- ➢ Eat healthy food
- ➢ Check your blood pressure/ cholesterol
- ➢ Exercise (get up and get moving)
- ➢ Manage blood sugar levels
- ➢ Quit smoking and drinking excessive alcohol
- ➢ Know your Body Mass Index (BMI)
- ➢ Sleep, Sleep, Sleep (the body needs to rest)
- ➢ Always schedule health screenings and vaccinations
- ➢ Mental health awareness

➢ Practice safe sex.

Improving the health of African Americans will take a lot more than community-based interventions. It will take self-discipline on the individual's part, dedication, and consistency to experience a major improvement in their health.

9

CHAPTER

PRECISION MEDICINE

African Americans haven't always been included in medical health research. Well, at least to their knowledge or consent. In the past, researchers would use black bodies in laboratory experiments, but never allow them to decide if they want to participant in clinical trials. Being included in health research means developing treatments that are personalized to the health needs of African Americans. When researchers exclude minorities from health research studies, it delays treatment, prevention, and effective care. Too often, health care is a one-size-fits all approach to medicine. Treatments meant for the average patient may not work well for individual people. African Americans have suffered from treatment (medication) that doesn't always work for their health needs. Instead of improving their health, these treatments often deteriorate their health because of the reaction to the medicine.

What is the Public Health Problem? The problem is disease and prevention strategies in healthcare haven't always considered an individual's genes, health history, environment, and lifestyle. African Americans are more likely to be more susceptible to disease depending on their family health history, environment, and their social lifestyle.

Which means not all treatment and prevention methods will work for this population. Individuals may suffer from unnecessary side effects from medications because of this one-size-fits-all approach for treatment. It's important for health professionals to consider everything that contributes to an individual's health.

Many healthcare professionals do not understand the importance of interpreting results from a genetic test. When interpreting a genetic test result, health care providers consider a person's medical history and family history. Knowing this information will make it easier for developing a treatment and prevention strategies specifically for the individual. Every patient is unique, and doctors need to tailor their treatments for the best results.

According to CDC, precision medicine—also called personalized medicine—"helps your doctor find your unique disease risks and treatments that will work best for you." In other words, precision medicine is an emerging approach to disease treatment and prevention that considers an individual's variability in genes, environment, and lifestyle for each person. Precision medicine allows doctors and researchers to create a personalized treatment plan for an individual based on a genetic knowledge of the patient's disease. This new evolving approach focuses on the root cause of the illness instead of addressing a patient's symptoms. It's important to note the environment affects the health of an individual and other populations. However, most health professionals don't always recognize the environment as a health risk factor.

Precision medicine will help improve health care through research. This will create more opportunities for researchers to understand the risk factors for certain illnesses and to figure out which treatment works best for people of different cultural backgrounds. Precision medicine means faster, efficient pathway towards a cure.

Precision medicine is the future for medicine because it gives physicians the tools to better understand the complex biological and environmental mechanisms of an individual's health and disease or condition. These innovations are leading to a transformation in cancer treatment, especially since there's a cancer disparity in the black community. As mentioned in earlier chapters, African Americans have the highest death rate and shortest survival of any racial/ethnic group for most cancers. Because of these advances with precision medicine, people with breast, lung, or colorectal cancers now routinely undergo molecular testing as part of their disease evaluation and treatment plan. These efforts may increase survival and reduce possible adverse effects for patients.

African Americans deserve a fair opportunity to be included in health research that can improve their health. Structural racism has been a major barrier in the healthcare system for African Americans for many years. It would be naive to believe that its impact would not affect the work that's being done into the field of precision medicine. The lack of inclusion, social disadvantage, and health disparities is a concern. However, precision medicine is a rare opportunity to bridge some of the long-standing racial gaps in health care and research. It's the solution for health disparities among African Americans in health care and research. It's a step in the right direction. It is a unique opportunity for medical researchers and physicians to correct the wrong of past distrust among black patients and researchers. The African American community, especially in the research field, has also been traumatized by a long history of exploitation, abuse, and marginalization. Precision medicine will hopefully open the door for African Americans to feel important in health research and know their health matters enough to develop a personalized treatment to improve it.

10
CHAPTER

HEALTH PROMOTION JOURNAL

"Taking care of myself doesn't mean me first, it means me too."

– L.R. Knost

Everyone feels differently every day. There are times you may experience pain in your body, feelings of sadness, or extreme fatigue that you haven't felt before. You also may not realize that these symptoms can be associated with an underlying condition or a serious disease. Knowing your health history is knowing your identity. Your family's history with health is a window to what may potentially be your health. With this information, preventive measures can be implemented in your life to end the cycle of unhealthiness and disease in your family.

What is your family health history?

....
....
....
....

Do you have any chronic diseases, such as heart disease or diabetes, or health conditions such as high blood pressure or high cholesterol?

....
....
....
....

How can I use my family health history to improve my health?

....
....
....
....

Has your mother or sister had breast cancer?

....
....
....
....

Does your parent or siblings have diabetes?

....
....
....
....

Did your parents or siblings get colorectal (colon) cancer before age 50?

....
....

....

....

Do you have any past medical problems?

....

....

....

....

Have you ever received medical care? If so, what problems/issues were addressed?

....

....

....

....

Have you ever smoked cigarettes? If so, how many packs per day and for how many years?

....

....

....

....

Do you drink alcohol? If so, how much per day and what type of alcohol do you consume?

....

....

....

....

Are you sexually active? Are you involved in a stable relationship?

....
....
....
....

Do you use condoms or other means of contraception?

....
....
....
....

Do you have a primary care physician (PCP)?

....
....
....
....

When was the last time you did a wellness check-up?

....
....
....
....

Do you keep your follow-up appointments?

....
....
....
....

Do you feel comfortable talking to your doctor about your health concerns?

....
....
....
....

Were you honest and accurate with your doctor?

....
....
....
....

What is your eating habit?

....
....
....
....

How often in one day do you eat fruits and vegetables?

....
....
....
....
....

Where is the nearest fresh food market in your area?

....
....

....
....
....

How often do you purchase fresh fruits and vegetables?

....
....
....
....

How do you feel today?

....
....
....
....
....

How often do you feel happy, sad, angry, or tired?

....
....
....
....

Do you have thoughts of suicide, harming yourself, or harming others?

....
....
....
....

Do you ever have thoughts that nothing in your life will change?

....

....

....

....

....

Do you feel depressed?

....

....

....

....

....

Do you have a support system or community you can confide in?

....

....

....

....

....

What have you done to today that brings you joy?

....

....

....

....

....

Write down your health goals:

....
....
....
....
....
....
....
....
....
....
....
....
....
....
....
....
....
....
....
....
....
....
....
....
....
....

REFERENCES

Center for Disease Control and Prevention. (2017). *Patterns and Trends in Age-Specific Black-White Differences in Breast Cancer Incidence and Mortality – United States, 1999–2014.* Retrieved from:
https://www.cdc.gov/mmwr/volumes/65/wr/mm6540a1.htm?CDC_AA_refVal=https%3A%2F%2Fwww

Center for Disease Control and Prevention. (2022). *Preventing Youth Violence.* Retrieved from
https://www.cdc.gov/violenceprevention/youthviolence/fastfact.html

Center for Disease Control and Prevention. (2022). *Precision health: Improving health for each of us and all of us.* Retrieved from
https://www.cdc.gov/genomics/about/precision_med.htm

Center for Disease Control and Prevention. (2022). *Disparities in Suicide.* Retrieved from
https://www.cdc.gov/suicide/facts/disparities-in-suicide.html

U.S. Department of Health and Human Services Office of Minority Health. (2021). *Mental and Behavioral Health - African Americans.* Retrieved from
https://www.minorityhealth.hhs.gov/omh/browse.aspx?lvl=4&lvlid=24

U.S. Department of Health and Human Services Office of Minority Health. (2021). Cancer and African Americans. Retrieved from
https://minorityhealth.hhs.gov/omh/browse.aspx?lvl=4&lvlid=16

American Cancer Society. (2022). *Cancer Disparities in the Black Community*. Retrieved from https://www.cancer.org/about-us/what-we-do/health-equity/cancer-disparities-in-the-black-community.html

American Cancer Society. (2022). American Cancer Society Guidelines for the Early Detection of Cancer. Retrieved from https://www.cancer.org/healthy/find-cancer-early/american-cancer-society-guidelines-for-the-early-detection-of-cancer.html

National Perinatal Association. (2018). *Free Resources.* Retrieved from https://www.nationalperinatal.org/resources/Documents/Position-Papers/2018-Position-Statement-PMADs_NPA.pdf

The Black Men's Health Project. (2022). *Rise In Health Today.* Retrieved from http://blackmenshealthproject.org/

American Psychiatric Association. (2022). *Diversity and Health Equity Education: African Americans-Mental Health Facts for African Americans.* Retrieved from https://www.psychiatry.org/psychiatrists/cultural-competency/education/african-american-patients

University of North Carolina. (2022). *Racism is an Adverse Childhood Experience (ACE)-The National Survey of Children's Health (NSCH).* Retrieved from https://ncchw.unca.edu/news-events/racism-is-an-adverse-childhood-experience-ace/

History. (2021). *Tuskegee Experiment: The Infamous Syphilis Study.* Retrieved from https://www.history.com/news/the-infamous-40-year-tuskegee-study

History. (2022). *The 'Father of Modern Gynecology' Performed Shocking Experiments on Enslaved Women.* Retrieved from https://www.history.com/news/the-father-of-modern-gynecology-performed-shocking-experiments-on-slaves

Johns Hopkins Medicine. (2022). *The Legacy of Henrietta Lacks-Honoring Henrietta.* Retrieved from https://www.hopkinsmedicine.org/henriettalacks/

American Progress. (2018). *Systematic Inequality.* Retrieved from https://www.americanprogress.org/article/systematic-inequality/

Healthy People. (2022). *Access to Health Services.* Retrieved from https://www.healthypeople.gov/2020/topics-objectives/topic/social-determinants-health/interventions-resources/access-to-health

Mayo Clinic. (2022). *Sickle Cell Anemia.* Retrieved from https://www.mayoclinic.org/diseases-conditions/sickle-cell-anemia/symptoms-causes/syc-20355876

Oak Street Health. (2021). *Diseases Affecting African Americans: Causes, Prevention, Etc.* Retrieved from https://www.oakstreethealth.com/diseases-affecting-african-americans-causes-prevention-etc-515308

www.ingramcontent.com/pod-product-compliance
Lightning Source LLC
Chambersburg PA
CBHW070028030426
42335CB00017B/2340